CHUG AND THUG

Ride Trike

By Gemal Seede, PhD

Illustrated by David Macedo

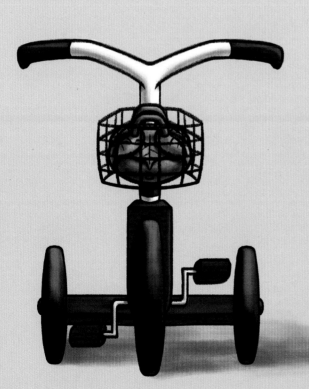

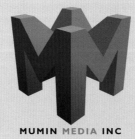

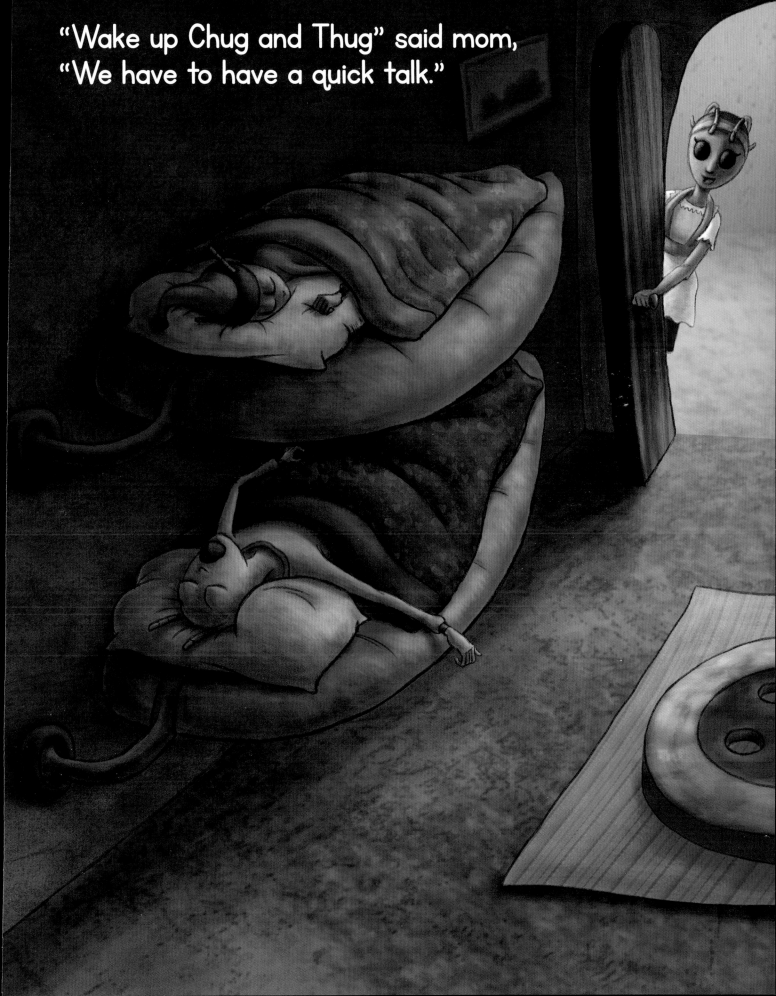

"Wake up Chug and Thug" said mom,
"We have to have a quick talk."

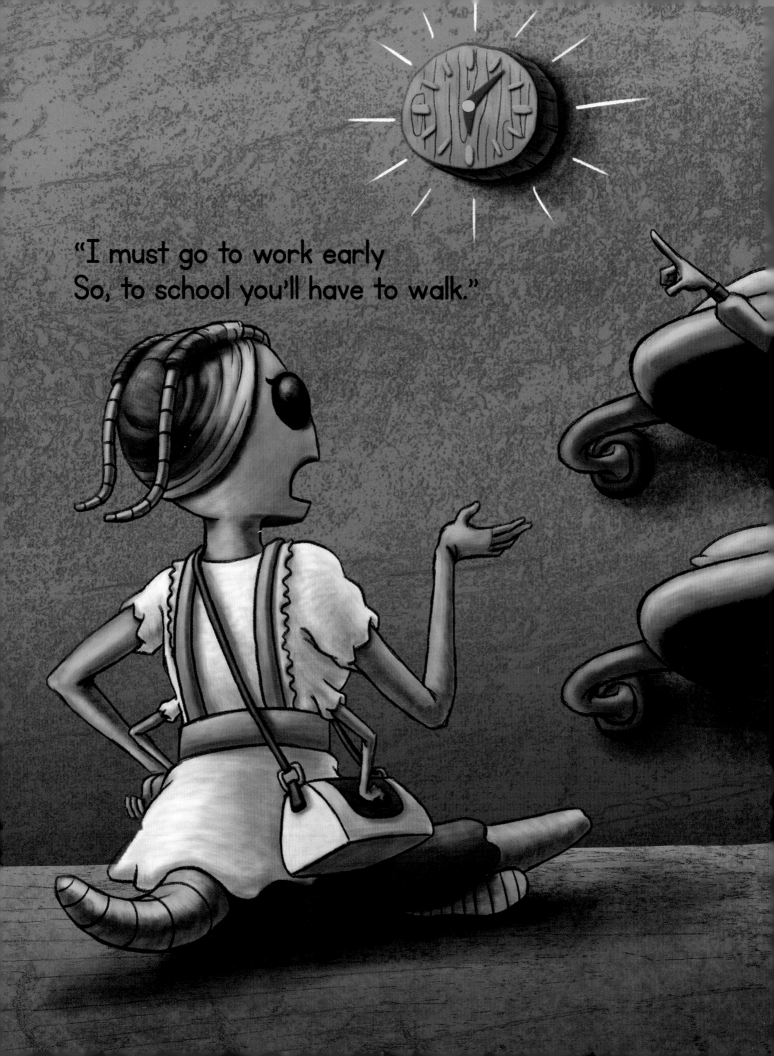

"I must go to work early
So, to school you'll have to walk."

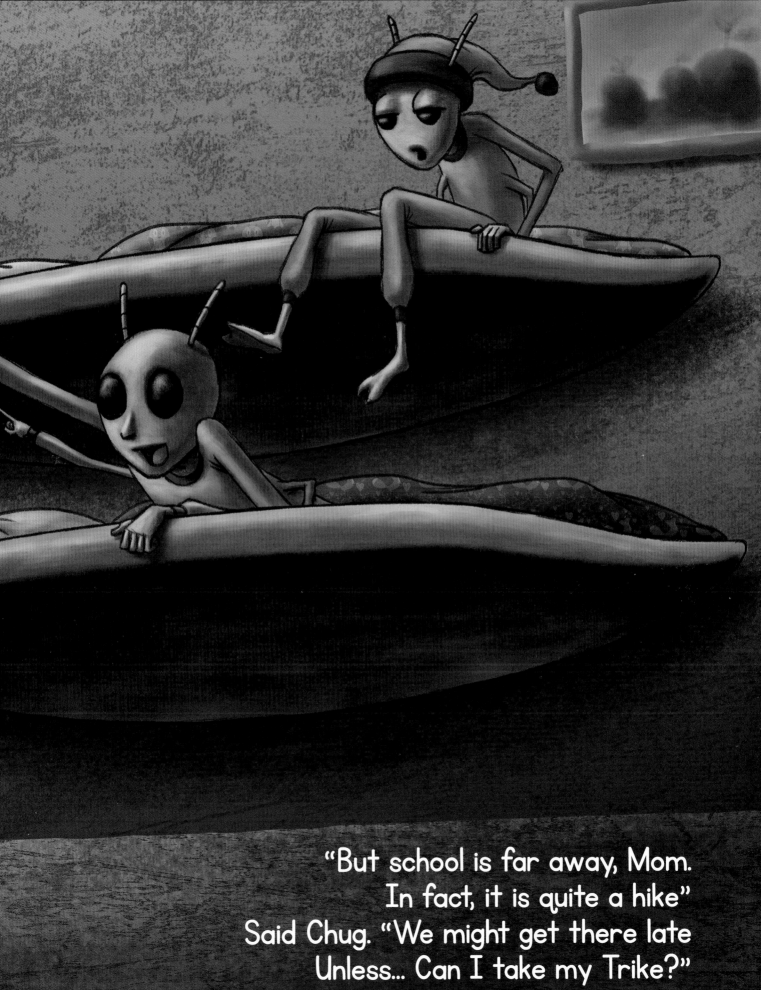

"But school is far away, Mom.
In fact, it is quite a hike"
Said Chug. "We might get there late
Unless... Can I take my Trike?"

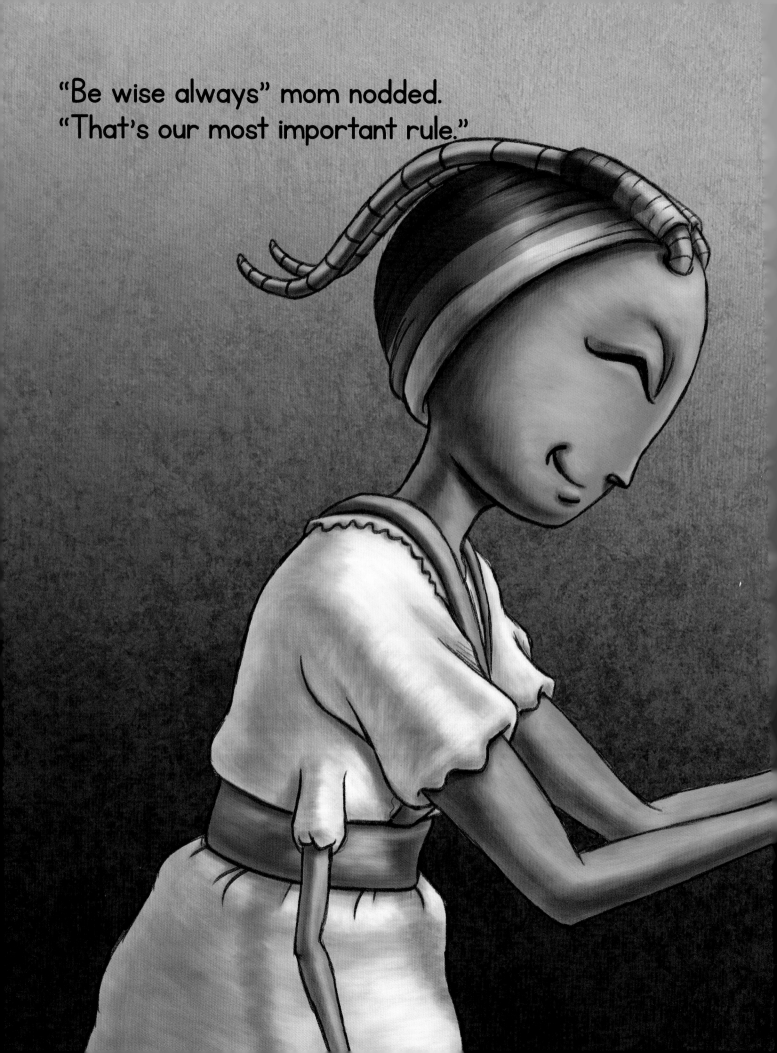

"Be wise always" mom nodded.
"That's our most important rule."

"Now hurry, hurry, hurry
Or you will be late for school."

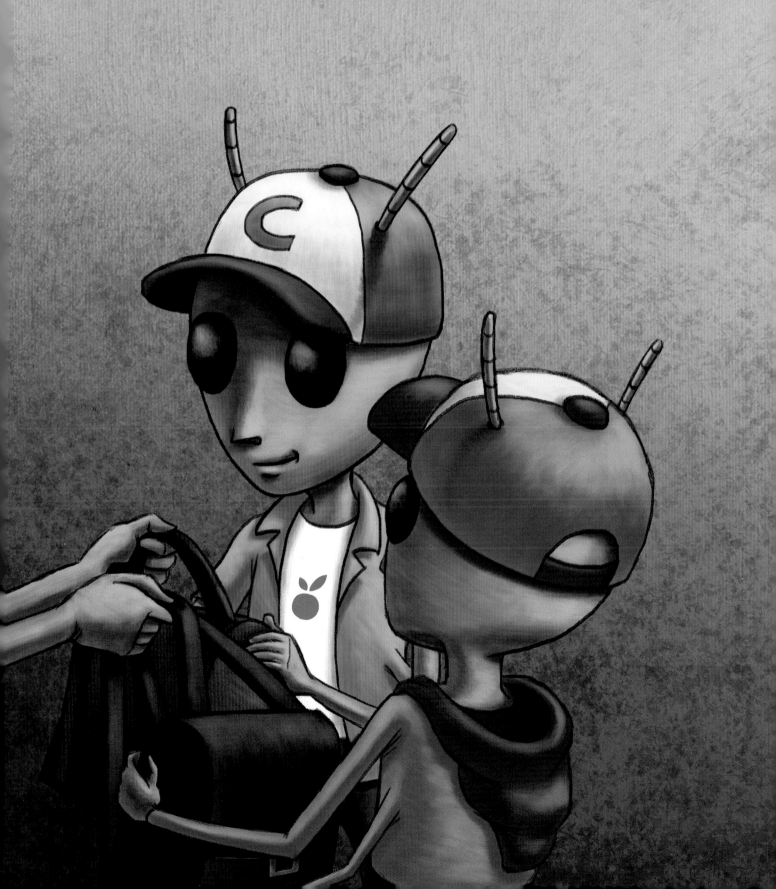

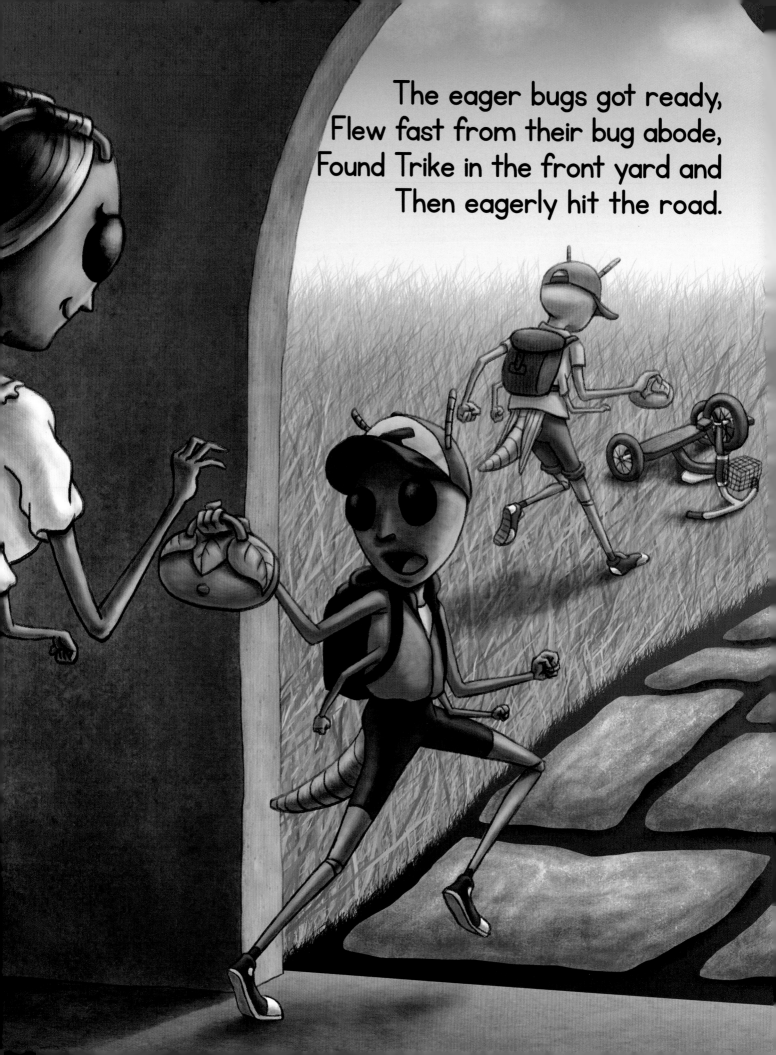

The eager bugs got ready,
Flew fast from their bug abode,
Found Trike in the front yard and
Then eagerly hit the road.

In front, Chug pumped the pedals.
Little Thug rode on the back.
The brothers were so happy
And they gave old Trike no slack.

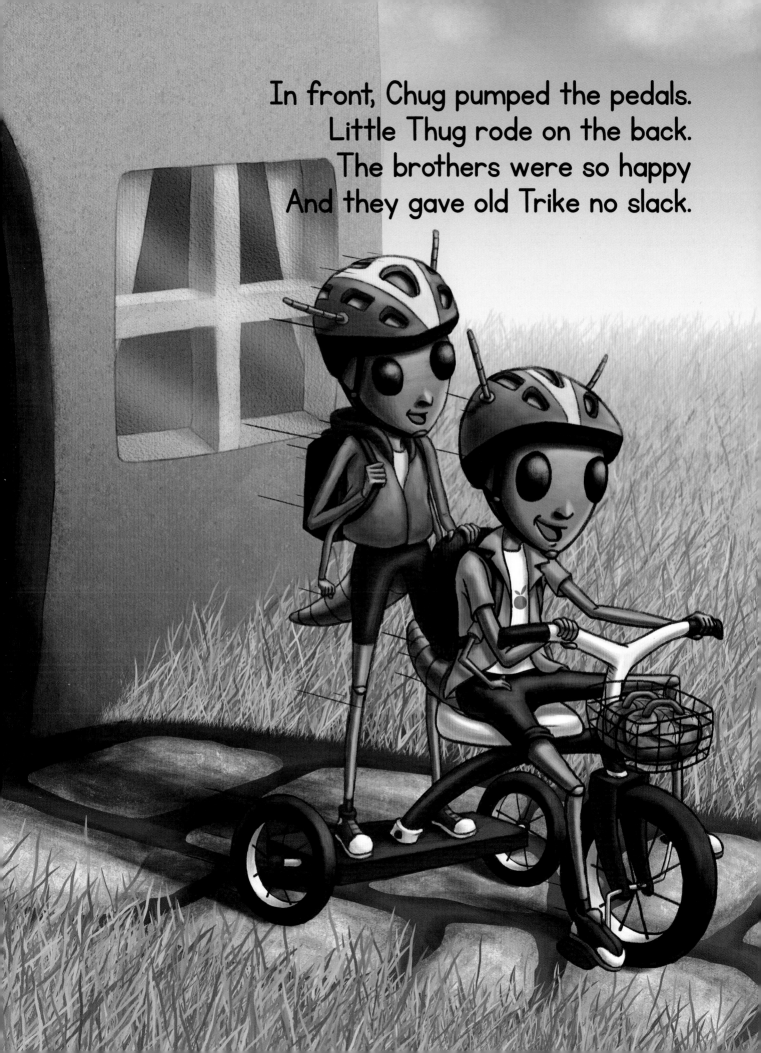

When they passed Sally Spider
She frowned and she shook her head.
The brothers did not know why
Until this is what she said.

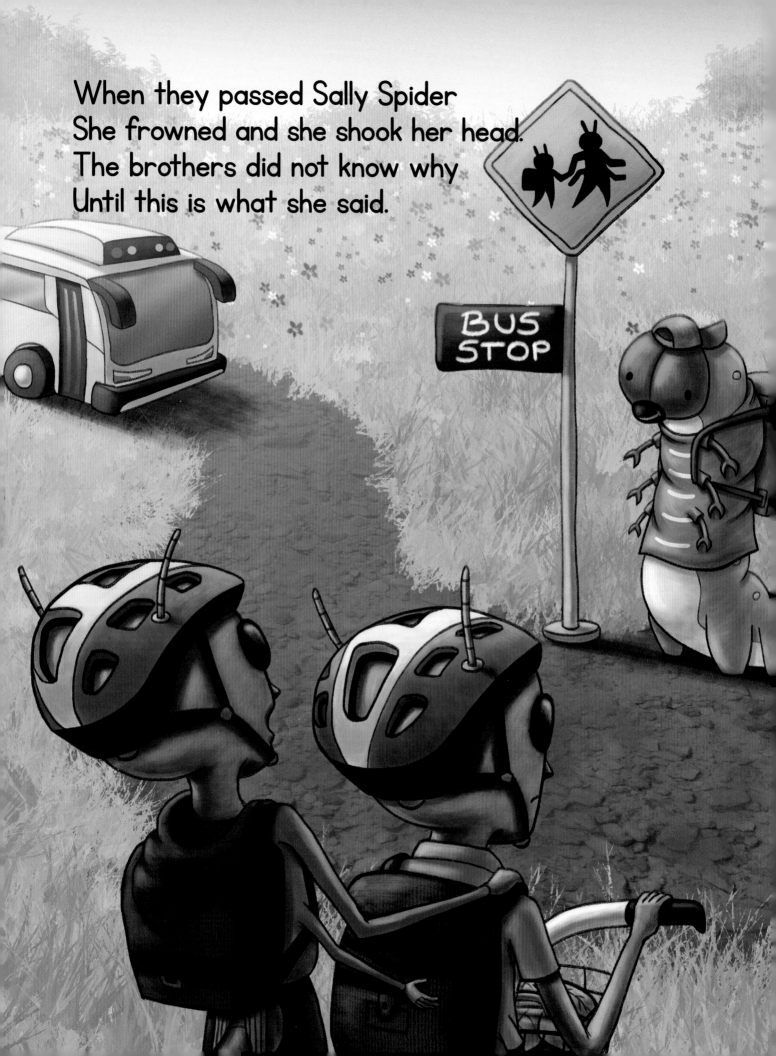

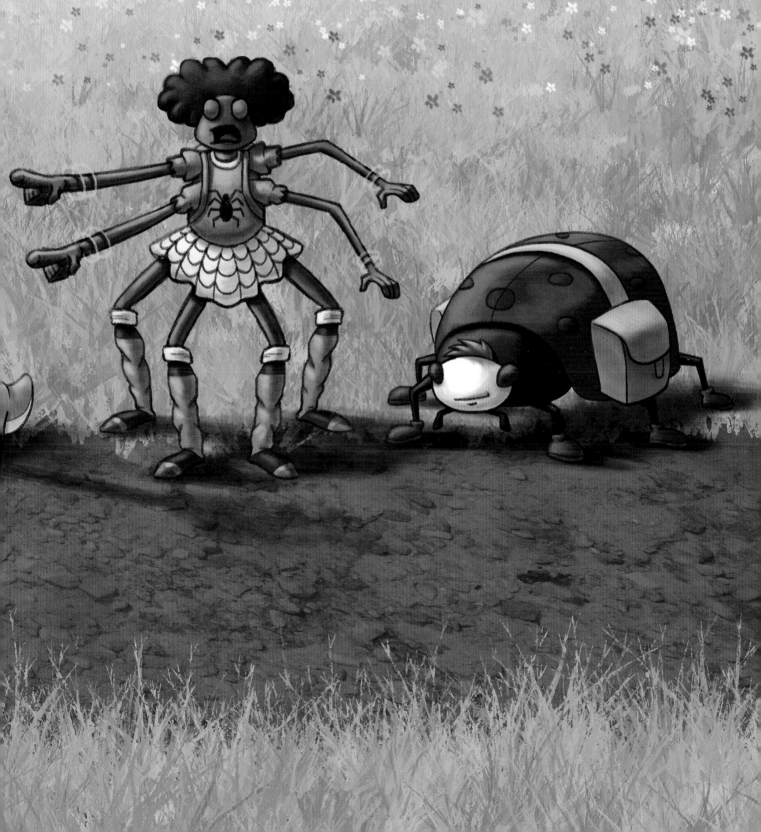

"Shame! Shame! Chug and Thug Alug.
Shame! Shame! For all goodness sake.
When you two ride on that Trike
Then that Trike you soon will break."

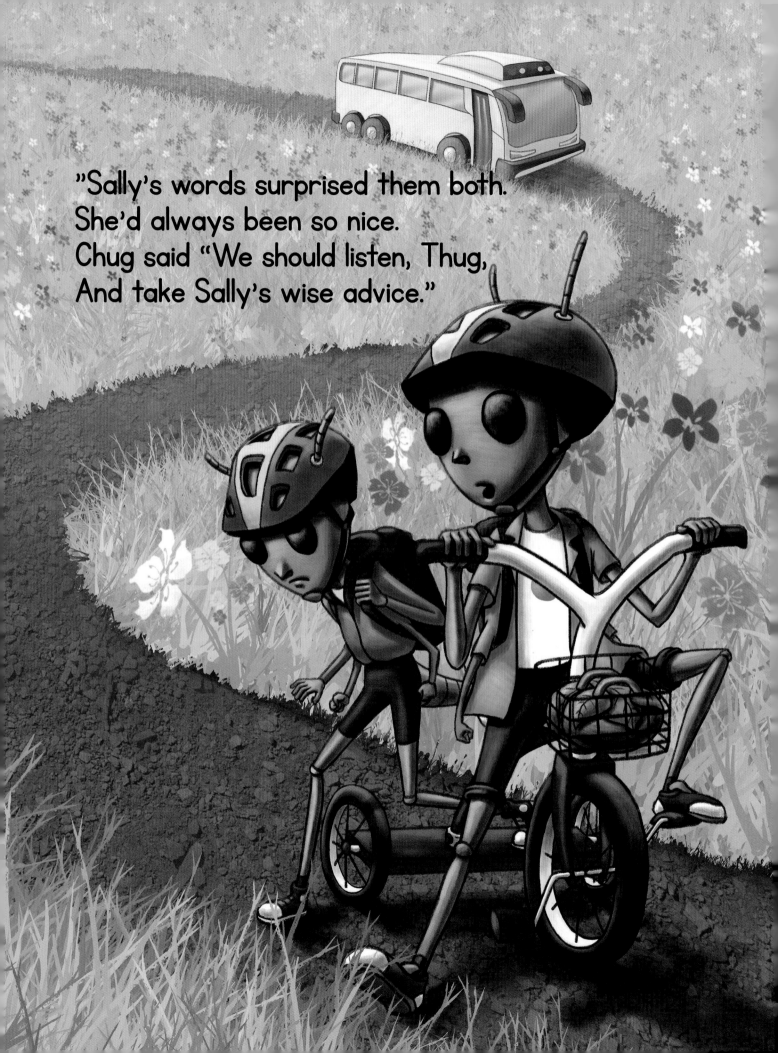

"Sally's words surprised them both.
She'd always been so nice.
Chug said "We should listen, Thug,
And take Sally's wise advice."

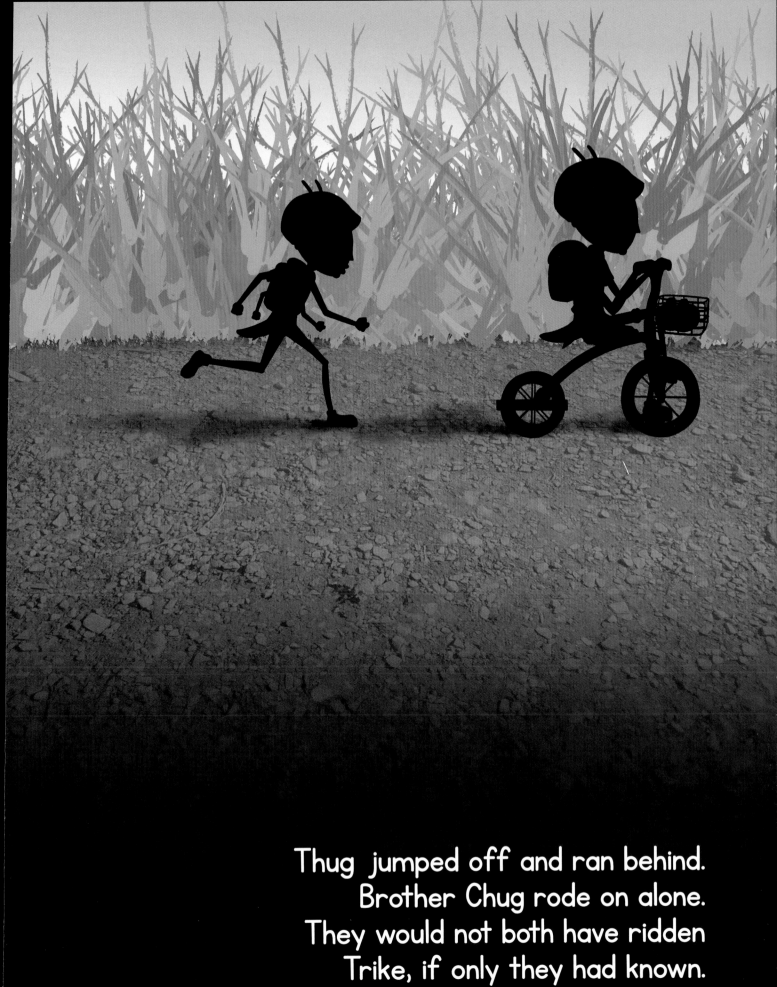

Thug jumped off and ran behind.
Brother Chug rode on alone.
They would not both have ridden
Trike, if only they had known.

Soon Worm Dude passed by. He was
Always mellow every place.
Yet something did upset him.
You could see it in his face.

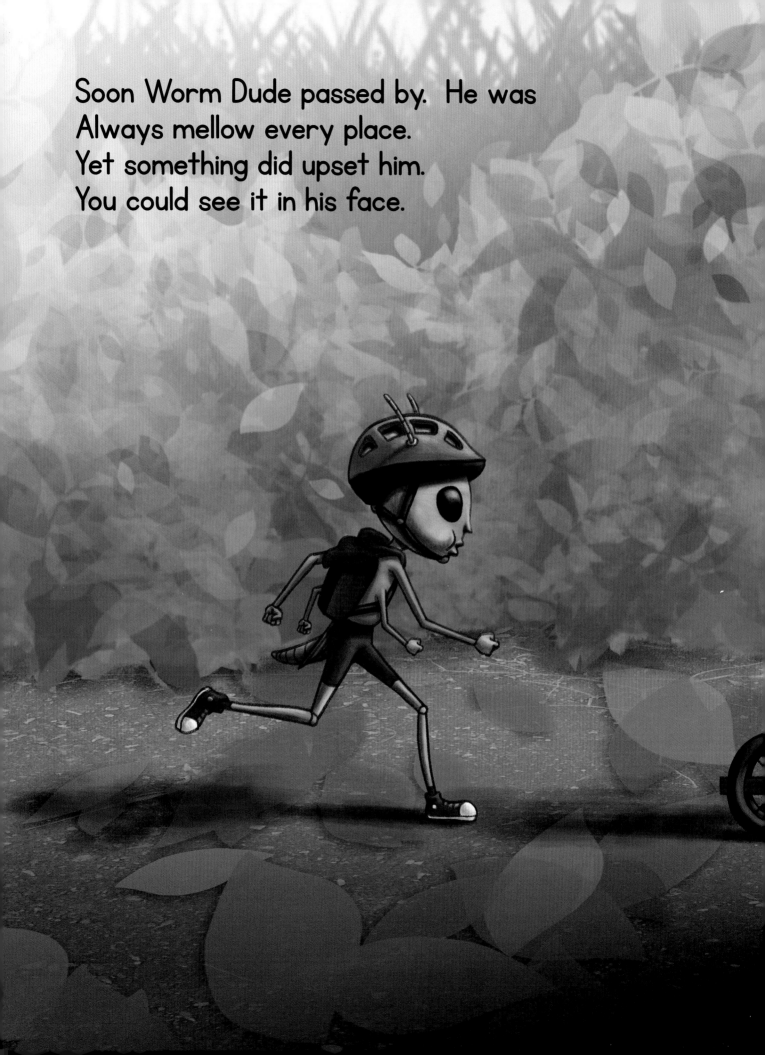

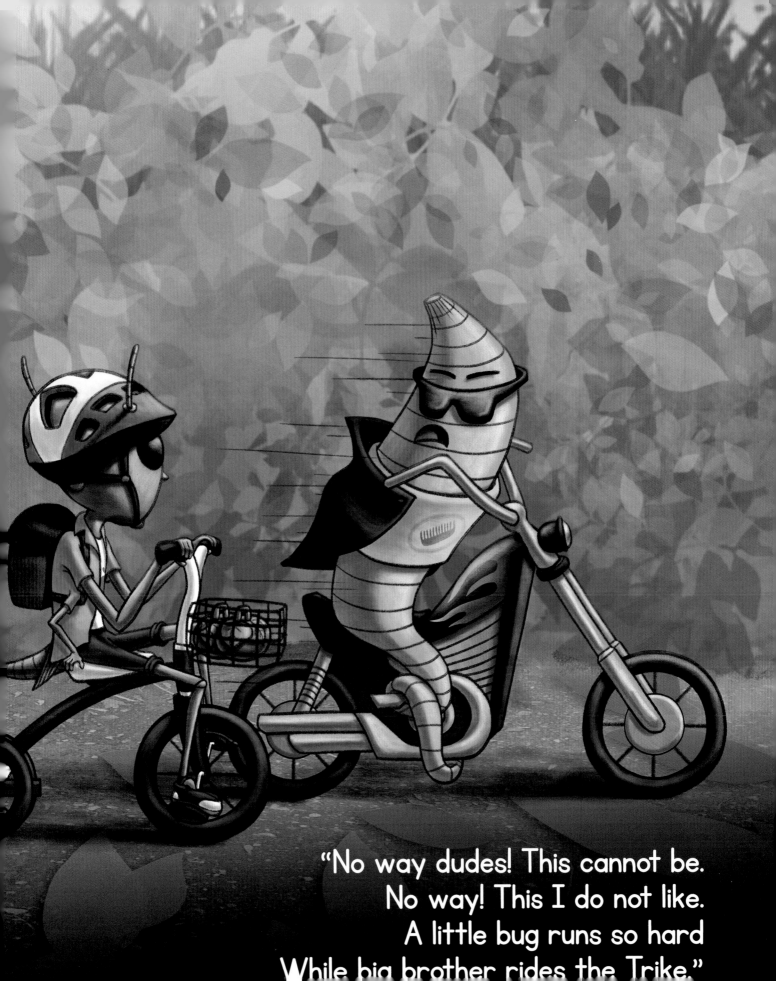

"No way dudes! This cannot be.
No way! This I do not like.
A little bug runs so hard
While big brother rides the Trike."

Worm Dude's words surprised them both
He'd always been so cool.
Chug said "I will listen, Thug,
And let you ride Trike to school."

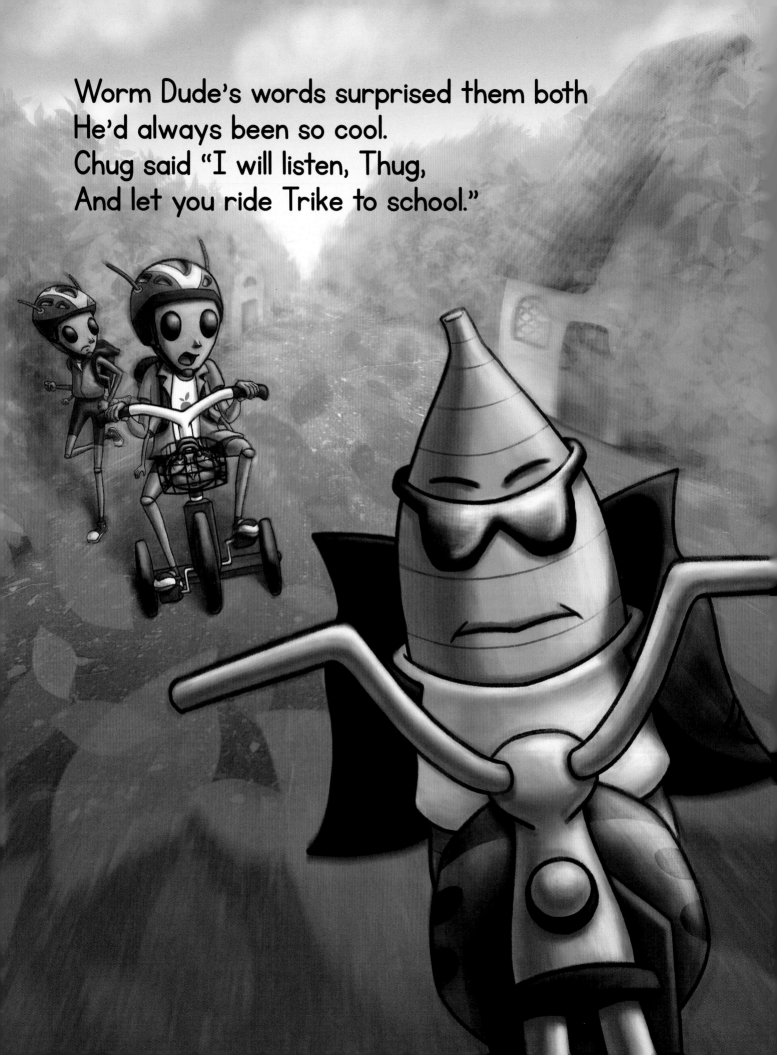

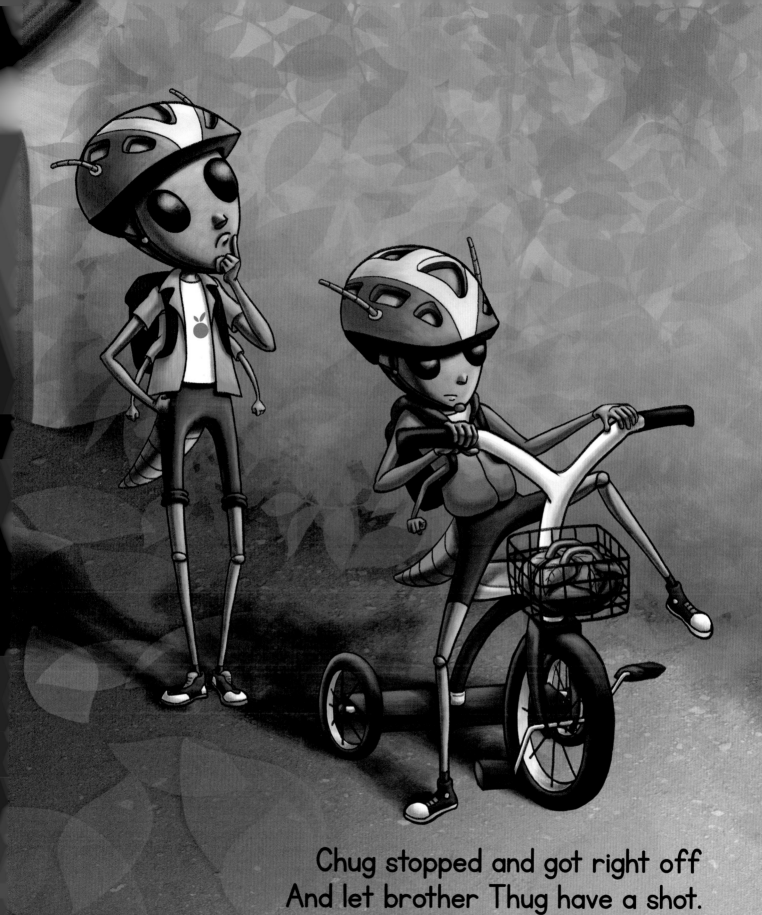

Chug stopped and got right off
And let brother Thug have a shot.
Chug wouldn't have been a selfish
Bug, if only he had thought.

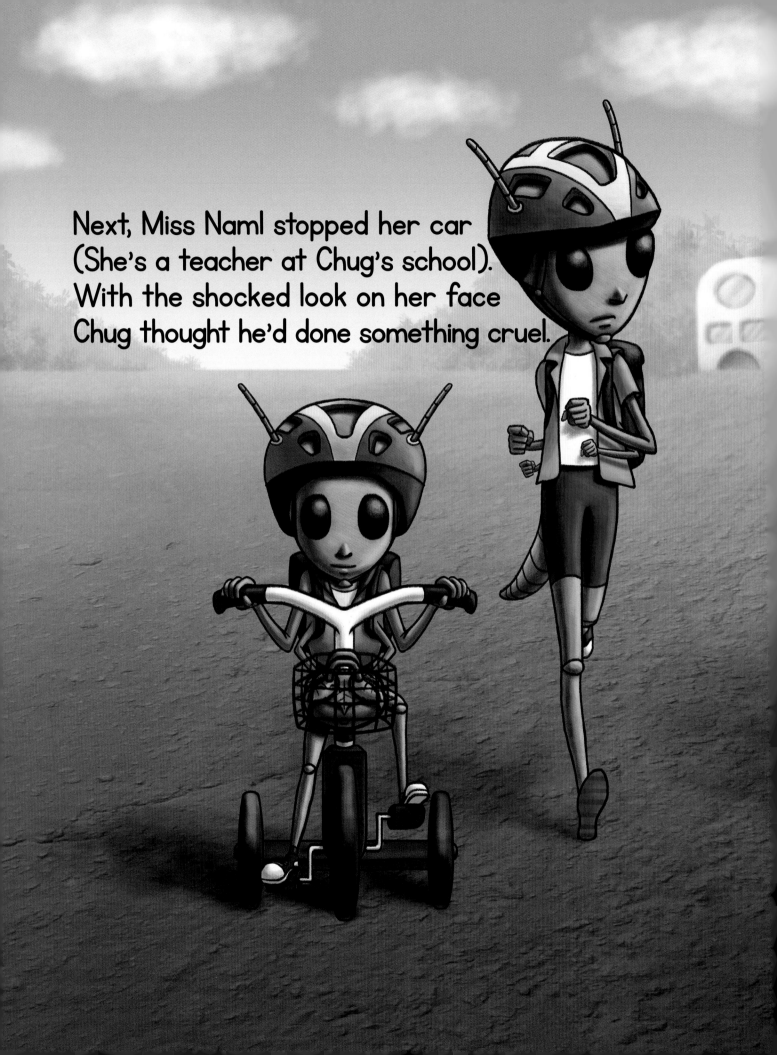

Next, Miss Naml stopped her car
(She's a teacher at Chug's school).
With the shocked look on her face
Chug thought he'd done something cruel.

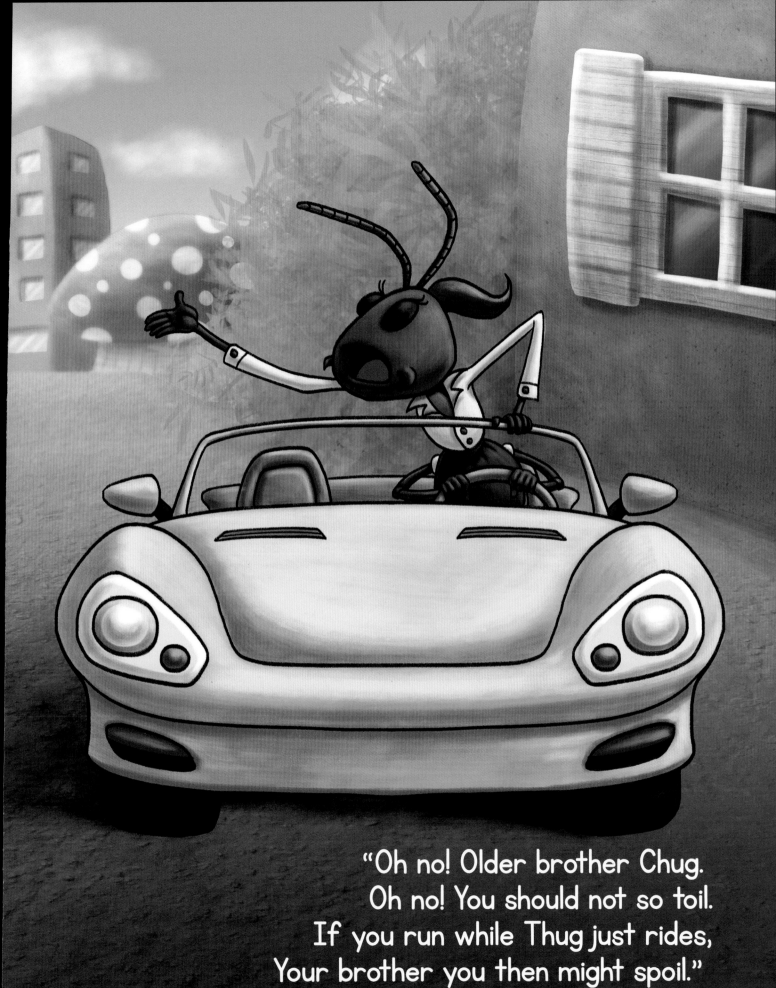

"Oh no! Older brother Chug.
Oh no! You should not so toil.
If you run while Thug just rides,
Your brother you then might spoil."

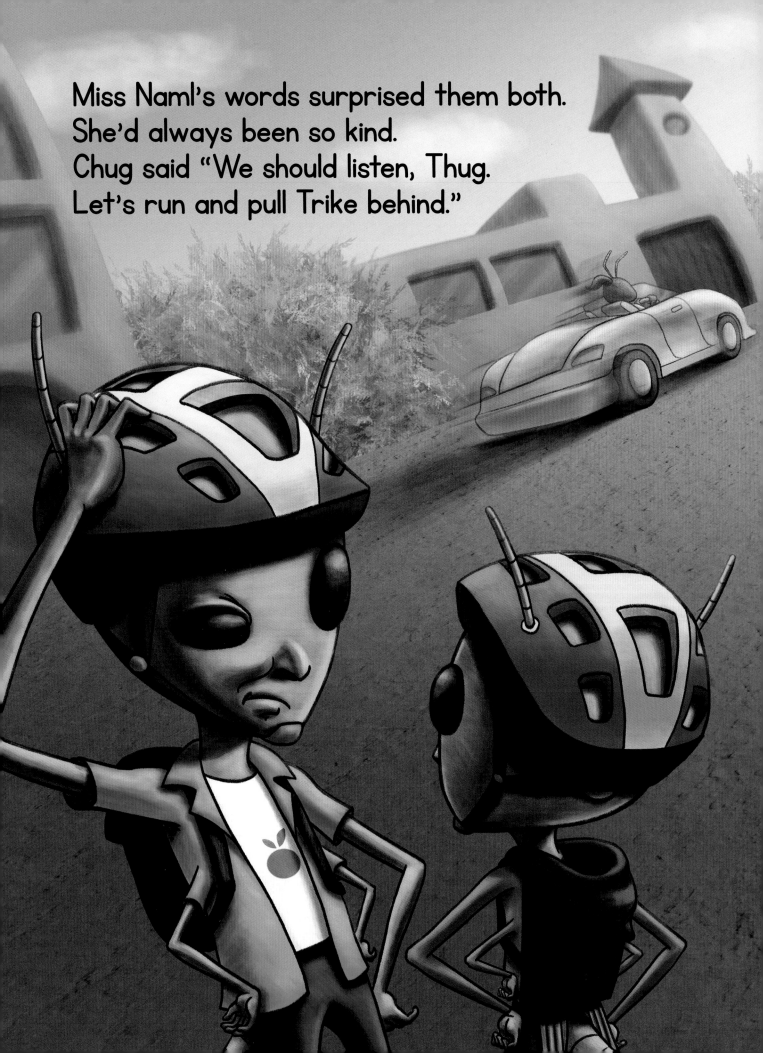

Miss Naml's words surprised them both.
She'd always been so kind.
Chug said "We should listen, Thug.
Let's run and pull Trike behind."

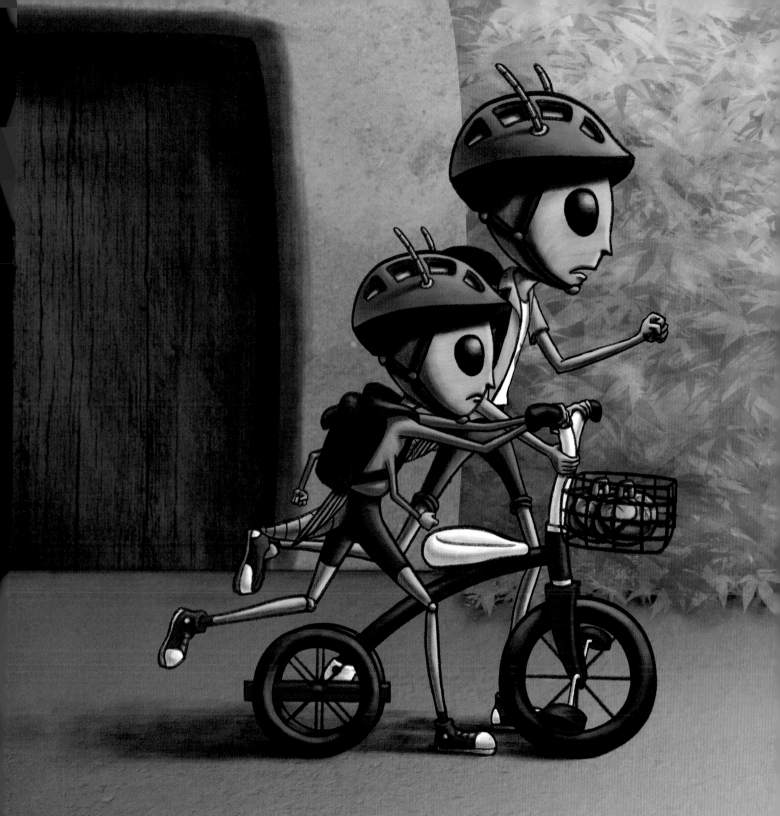

So, Chug climbed off. Both bugs ran
Pulling Trike as fast as they could.
Chug wouldn't have spoiled little Thug
If only he'd understood.

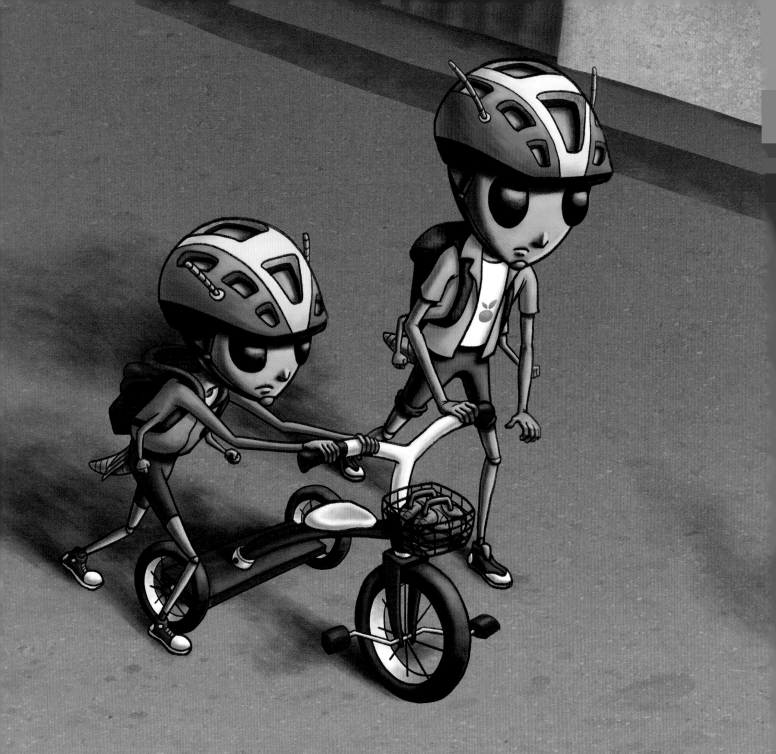

There old Hector Hornet stood
Watching Chug and Thug run past
Dragging little Trike behind.
The older bug was aghast.

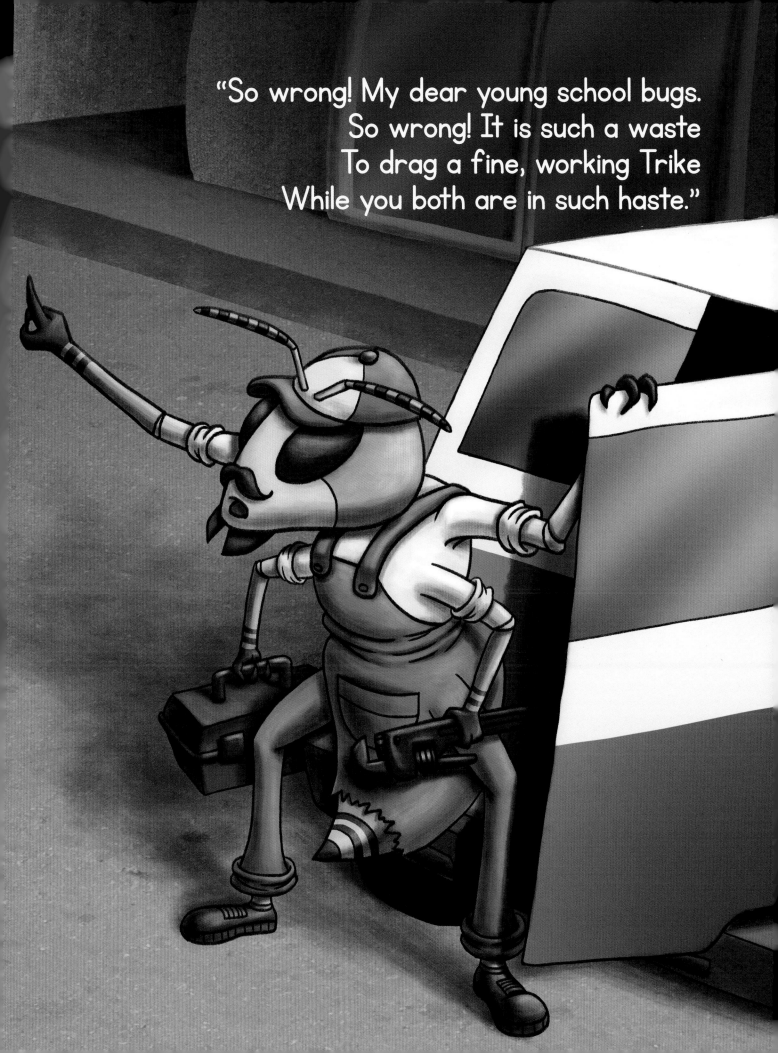

"So wrong! My dear young school bugs.
So wrong! It is such a waste
To drag a fine, working Trike
While you both are in such haste."

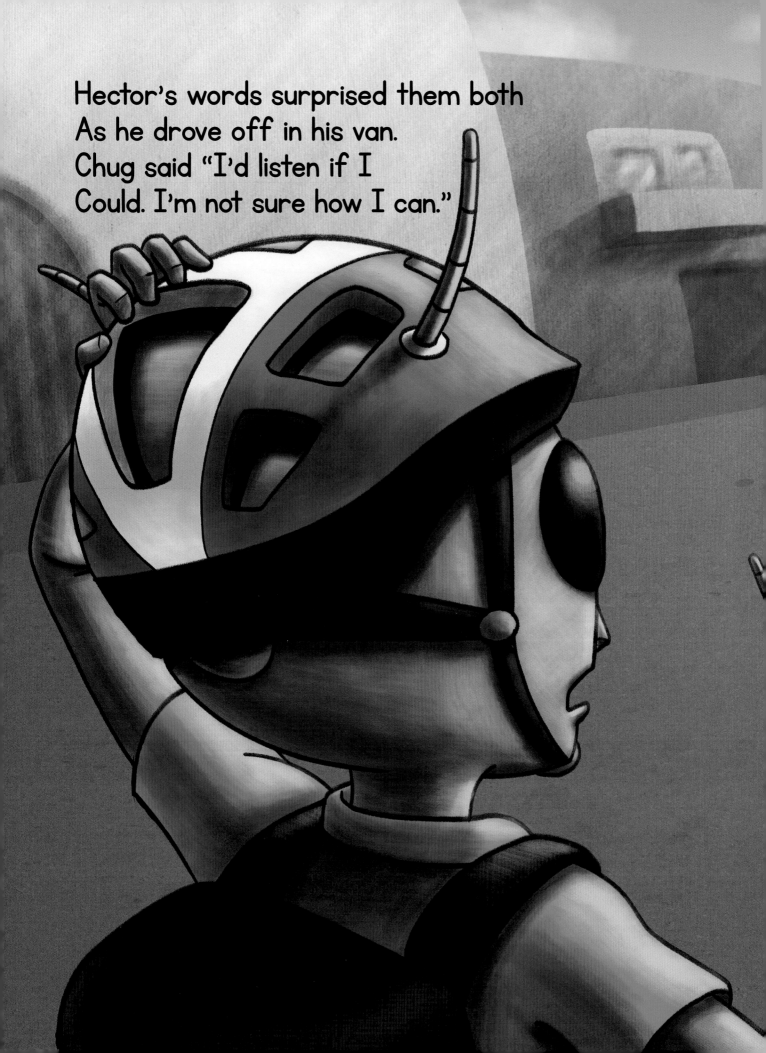

Hector's words surprised them both
As he drove off in his van.
Chug said "I'd listen if I
Could. I'm not sure how I can."

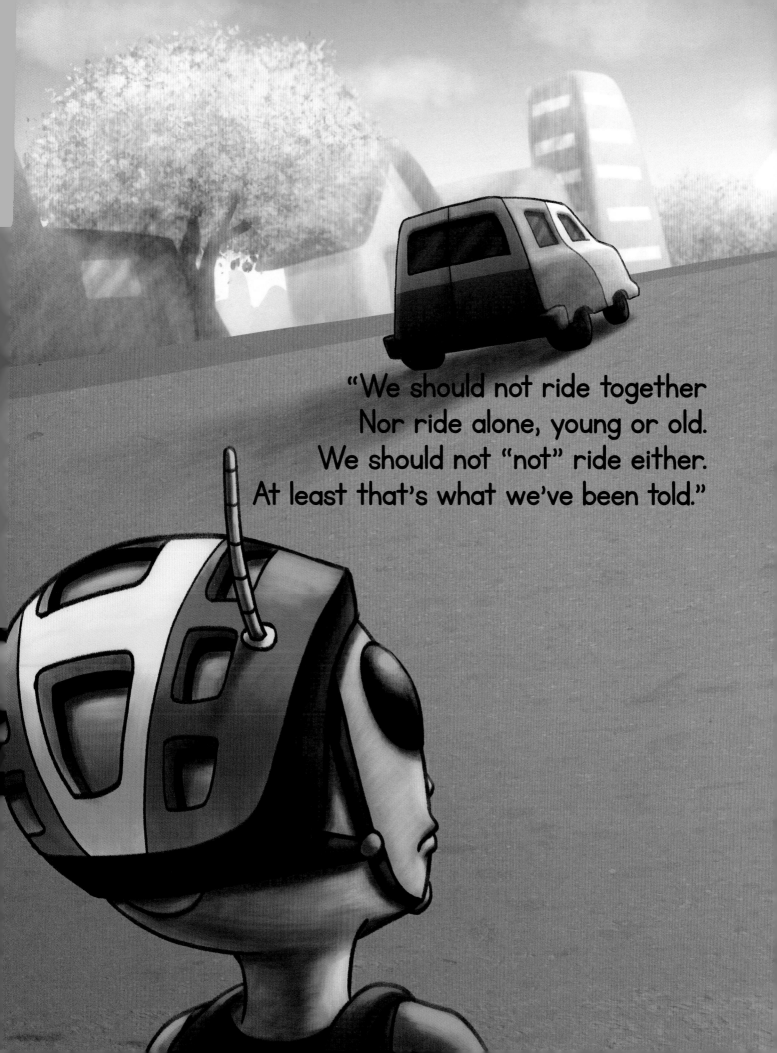

What to do now, the bugs thought?
The brothers were now quite stumped.
"I think we are stuck right here"
Said Chug as Thug's shoulders slumped.

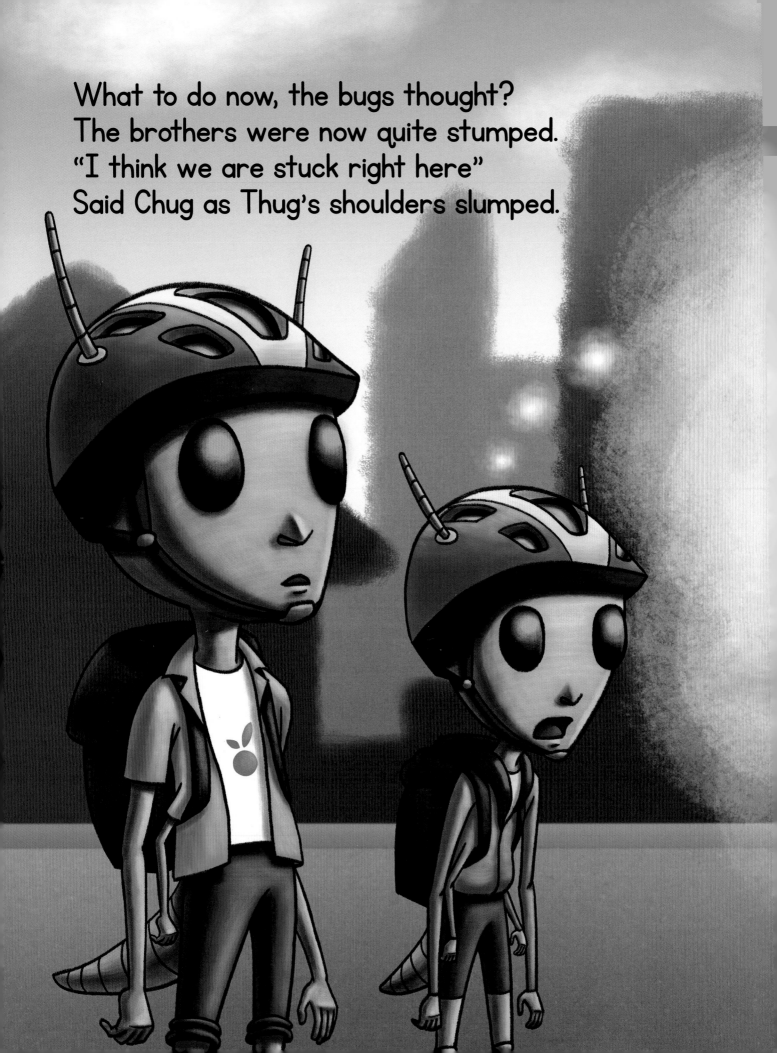

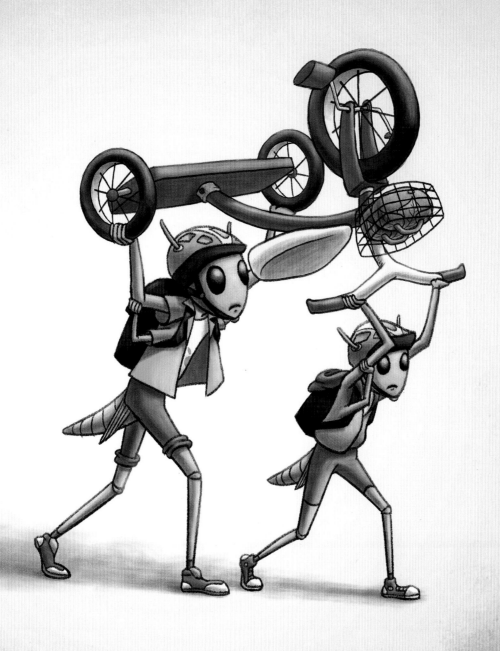

"We could carry Trike," sighed Thug
"Though we will be late for school."

Chug thought and thought.

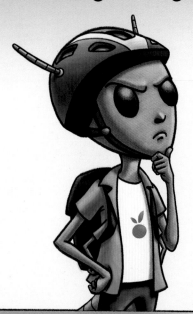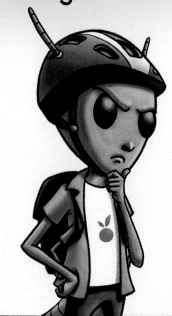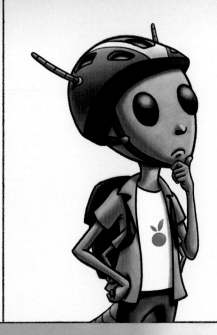

Then he laughed
"Oh Thug, I shan't be a fool.

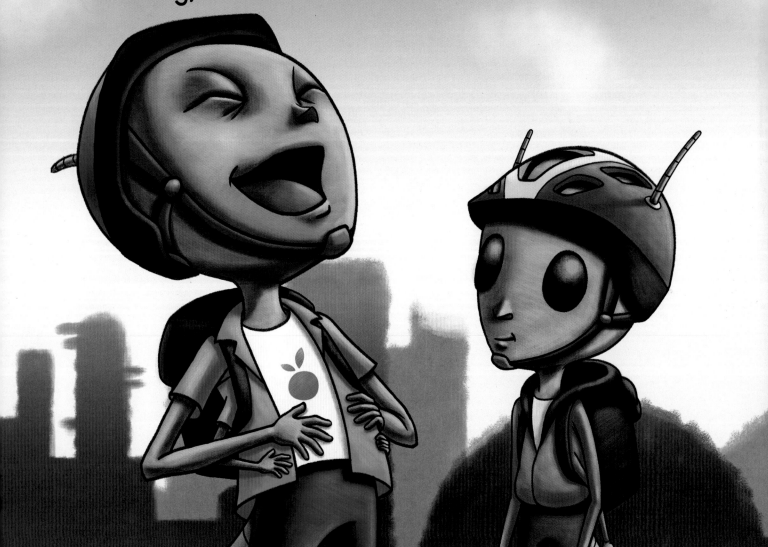

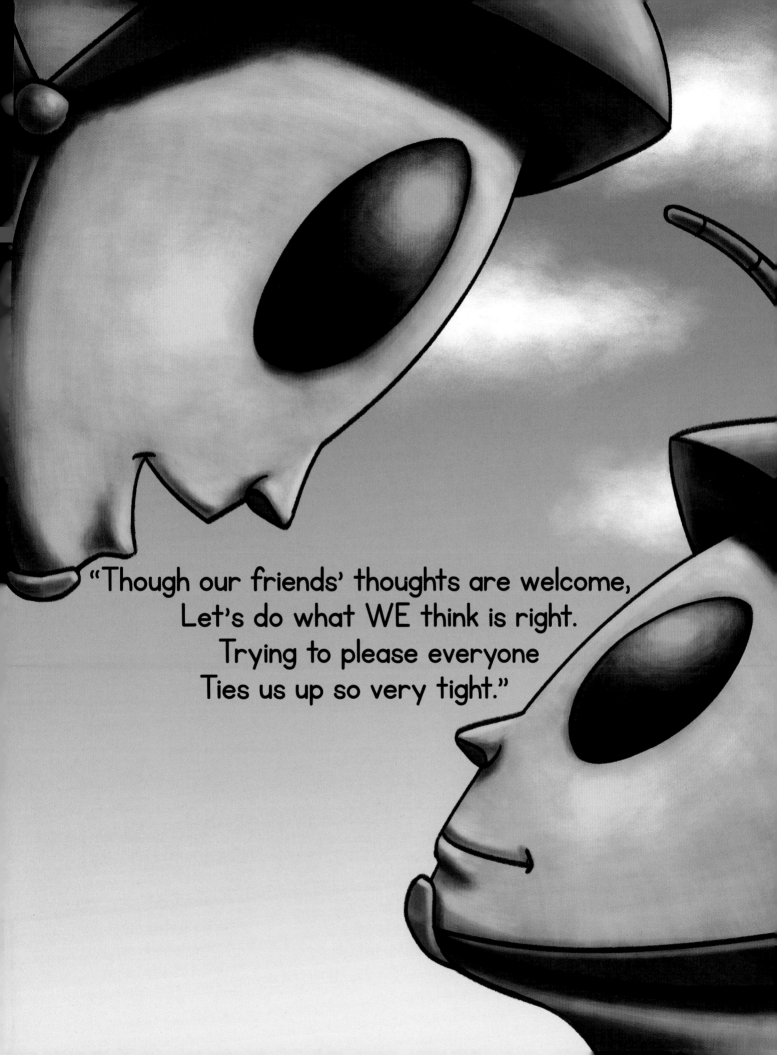

"Though our friends' thoughts are welcome,
Let's do what WE think is right.
Trying to please everyone
Ties us up so very tight."

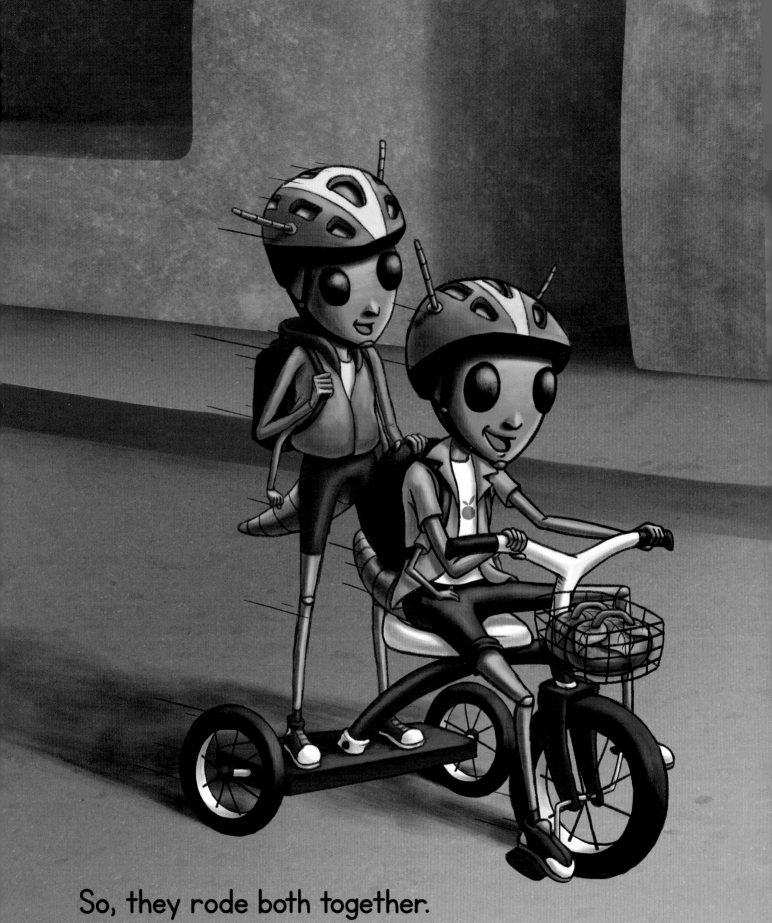

So, they rode both together.

Then sometimes each took a turn.

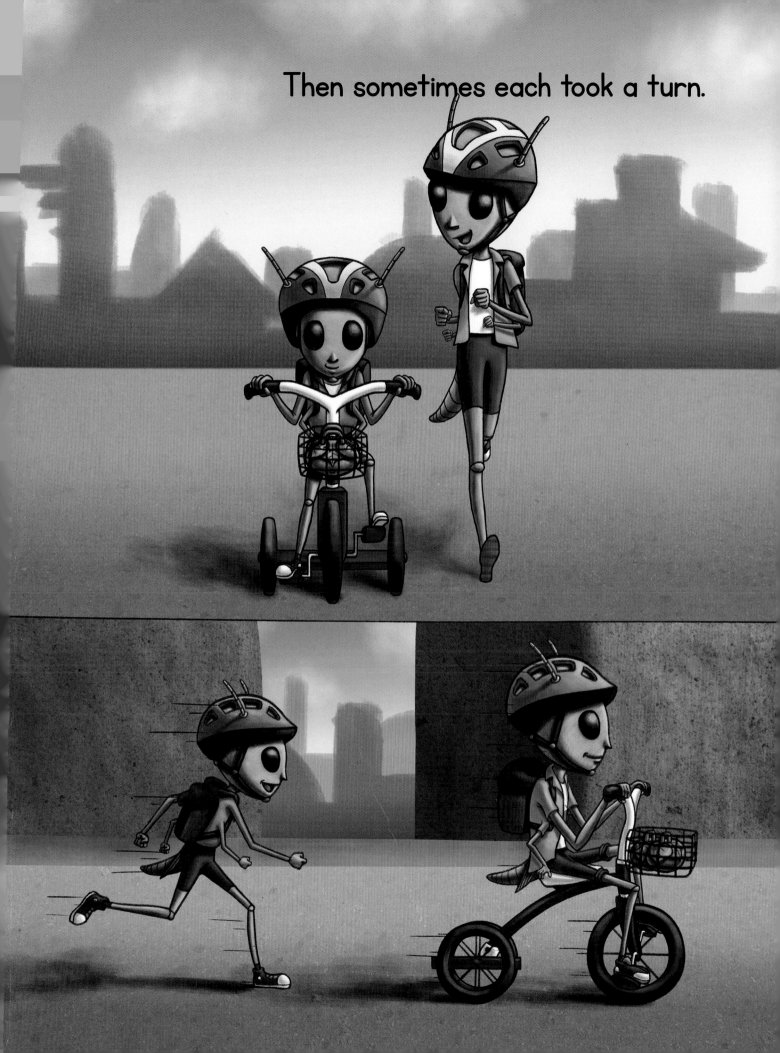

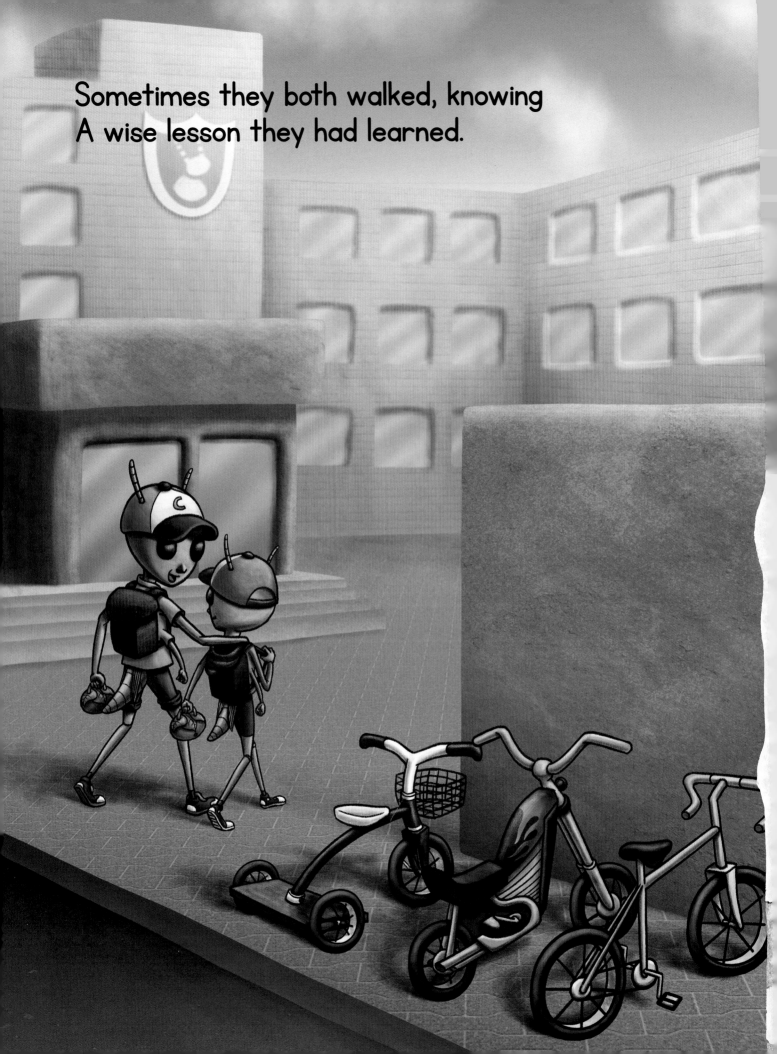

Sometimes they both walked, knowing
A wise lesson they had learned.

NOTE TO PARENTS AND TEACHERS

Chug and Thug Ride Trike is a fun adaptation of an oft-told fable common to many cultural traditions about a man, his son and his donkey. The earliest known written form of that story is by the 13th-century Arab writer Ibn Said al Maghribi, but the story is now included in many collections including the ancient Greek Aesop's tales.

Children sometimes do not voluntarily talk about emotional issues they face outside the home or classroom. Chug and Thug Ride Trike is a way to start a conversation with children about potential social or peer pressure that they may face, and gives them a way to think about them.

After reading this story with them, here are some suggested questions to ask your child:

- Did Chug and Thug's friends mean well? Did they believe the advice they gave Chug and Thug was good?
- Was the advice that Chug and Thug received helpful?
- Is it always possible to take everyone's advice? If not, how should kids decide on when to take advice from other people?
- Have you ever been in the same bind that Chug and Thug were in where people tried to convince you to do something and you thought it was not the best thing to do? What did you do?

I sincerely hope you and your child enjoy this story.

Best wishes,
Gemal Seede

For more information about this book, the author, the illustrator or the Chug and Thug book series, visit www.chugandthug.com

For more information about Mumin Books or its parent company, Mumin Media, visit www.mumin.media or www.muminmedia.ca